90

Days to Health

Body, Soul & Spirit Plan

Dr. C. Thomas Anderson

Winword
publishing house

Phoenix, Arizona

SECOND EDITION

Winword Publishing 2006 —
90 Days to Health, Body, Soul & Spirit Plan/
Dr. C. Thomas Anderson.—
Second Edition
ISBN 1-58588-099-X

Published by: Winword Publishing House
3520 East Brown Road
Mesa, AZ 85213

To order or for more information, contact us at:

(480) 985-6156

or visit: www.winwordpublishing.com

Table of Contents

Preface

A story is told of an overweight man who visited the doctor for a check up. The doctor told him, "You're going to have to give up those intimate dinners for two—until you find somebody to share them with."

It is troubling in a faith church to see how often people are affected by ill health. I believe that God has the power to heal anything and that He wants to heal every sickness. I have seen miracles happen, people healed from cancer, leukemia and tumors. I have seen people walk out of wheelchairs. I have seen others healed from virtually every kind of sickness this world has to offer. There is no question that God can heal. I have seen it too many times to believe otherwise. I have experienced it myself.

Yet I have also seen many people, some of them good friends, die before their time from sickness and disease. I have seen some that were good, born again, Spirit-filled, faith-believing Christians, go to be with the Lord before their time. I have seen many struggle with infirmities that they just can't seem to get over. And it troubles my heart.

America has devoted more time and money to the pursuit of health than any nation in history, yet so many of us have seemed to ignore the information available and our health has degenerated as a result. I believe that if we are to overcome the health problems that nag so many in the church we must learn to understand some things about our bodies. We need to become nutritionally literate.

The purpose of this study is to answer some of the questions about why faith people still get sick, and to find a biblical balance between the power of healing and the biblical principles of nutrition. I believe that God will heal you when you are sick. But I also believe that God will work through doctors and He will work through nutrition. He will heal you when you need it but He prefers to keep you healthy so that a miracle is not needed. There is much we can learn about how to live our lives and what kind of nutritional content we take in.

This is not an easy subject to teach. When I talk about health, it is easy for you to take in all the information and begin to believe that if you just eat certain things and take the right vitamins, you will automatically have health.

But you must never make health or health products or nutrition your god. You must never lose sight of the fact that health comes from God. One of the names of God is *Jehovah-Rapha'*. We usually translate it as "Jehovah who heals you" but literally it is "Jehovah who is your health." The process of keeping you healthy is just as much the work of God as healing you after you are sick. Even in discussing nutrition we can never get away from the power of faith.

We must meditate on the Word. We must speak the Word. We must see health. We must say health. We must live by the Word for health. Faith has the power to heal your physical body and to overcome any sickness and any disease. The grace of God has the power to overcome our weakness and imperfection. Health comes from God, not from vitamins.

With that in mind we are going to look at the way God made us. Your body was designed to respond to some things better than others. The Bible tells us a great deal about what God's perfect diet is. Put very simply, we can eat anything we want. It has been the tendency of the church for the last two thousand years to create religious rules derived from the misreading of scripture and completely miss the point of what God is trying to tell us.

Timothy was overseeing a church in Ephesus that was surrounded by religious thinking. Ephesus was the sight of the Temple of Diana, one of the architectural wonders of the ancient world. There was every kind of religious practice that could be imagined in that city from pagan sacrifices and temple prostitution to Greek philosophy and the worship of reason. When Paul wrote to Timothy he said many things that make it obvious that the people of Ephesus loved religion and they loved religious rules. It is also obvious that the attitudes permeated the church there as well. For example, Paul warned Timothy about those

> . . . *forbidding to marry, and commanding to abstain from foods which God created to be received with thanksgiving by those who believe and know the truth.* (1 Timothy 4:3)

There is not room here to discuss the history of the church's attitudes toward marriage. Many of the religious notions about marital relationships have had an impact on the family unit and it has not always been good. There was a time in history when church leaders encouraged men to leave their wives and children to fend for themselves, while they went off into the desert to become spiritual. The Bible makes it clear that the family is the most important earthly relationship there is and that a man who fails to care for his family is worse than an infidel. But that is another issue. For now we must focus on the comments about food.

Paul also addresses those who believe that Bible nutrition is all about what you can't eat. They see nutrition as a list of rules that dictate their diet. However, Paul goes on to tell Timothy that all food is good.

> . . . *commanding to abstain from foods which God created to be received with thanksgiving by those who believe and know the truth. For every creature of God is good, and nothing is to be refused if it is received with thanksgiving; for it is sanctified by the word of God and prayer.*
> (1 Timothy 4:3-5)

In other words, God said that we can eat anything we want. Every creature of God is good. When He created for six days, He looked at what He had made and He said it was good—all of it. There wasn't anything that wasn't good.

I should point out that it means everything that was food was good. There are some things that are not meant to be food that are not good for us. Arsenic, for example, is not good to eat. But everything that God considers food is good.

We need to recognize, however, that some foods are better than others. The problem is not what we eat. The problem is what we don't eat. The things we do eat often don't have all of the nutritional elements we need but they fill us up and then we never eat the foods that we do need.

There is nothing wrong with eating a donut. But if I have donuts for breakfast, donuts for lunch, donuts for dinner and donuts for a late night snack, and never eat anything else, I will starve my body to death. It is not the donuts that will kill me, it is the lack of essential nutrition. I will not get the necessary nutrients to keep my body running properly.

We need to learn what foods are best for us so that we provide our bodies with everything they need. This is not a religious idea. It is common sense. If you keep on eating nothing but donuts, it will not keep you from going to heaven. In fact it will probably help you get there sooner.

Most diseases and sicknesses are food related. But the problem is not what's in the food but rather what is not in the food. God designed the human body to resist and defeat virtually every kind of disease that there is, but it needs to be functioning at its full capacity to be able to do that. When we starve ourselves of proper nutrition we make it that much more difficult for our bodies to keep up. As a society, the things we eat make us fat but we are still starving and as a result we get sick.

This does not negate the miracle working power of God. None of us are perfect and we all have occasions when we are confronted with sickness. We walk in faith, knowing that God can and will heal us of every infirmity.

But God's design is to **keep** us healthy, not **make** us healthy. We understand repentance as turning away from sin but it also involves turning away from foolish living, including foolish nutrition. If we insist on not eating well, then we will need healing that much more.

Romans 2:5-7 talks about those who have a hard and impenitent heart. God "will render to each one according to his deeds" (verse 6). If you continually insist on starving your body, there will be problems. It's not that you have to get sick but your persistence in not providing your body with the nutrition it needs will cause it to eventually break down.

In Ephesians, Paul talked about putting on the armor of God.

Therefore take up the whole armor of God, that you may be able to withstand in the evil day, and having done all, to stand. (Ephesians 6:13)

We are to do all. That means all that we know to do. When we are sick, we know first of all that God can heal. But that does not mean that we should avoid doctors. Availing ourselves of their knowledge and training is part of doing all. Proper exercise to keep ourselves fit is part of doing all. Gaining nutritional literacy so that we stay as healthy as we can is also part of doing all.

It's not that God can't heal you. He can. He wants to. The problem is in our persistence in treating our bodies in ways God never intended. We need to learn how to eat intelligently so that we can live the way God planned for us to live. Healing is better than sickness but health is better than healing.

Introduction

We have much written about spiritual growth. We have hundreds of new books every month teaching us how to grow and mature in Christ. Likewise, there are hundreds of books on the market helping us to understand the mind, emotions, and the realm of the soul. There are also many books written about nutrition and the importance of vitamins, minerals and exercise. Good health requires a balanced knowledge in all of these areas. It also requires wisdom.

This book is a "how to," "how much," and "why" book concerning these three topics: spiritual well-being, emotional well-being, and physical well-being. While it is true that there is a great deal of knowledge circulating about these very important topics, sadly, there is not much understanding and very little wisdom accompanying this knowledge.

The Bible says that knowledge is the beginning of the fear of the Lord. However, God also warns us that knowledge can puff us up and make us prideful. Knowledge is only the beginning. Wisdom is the goal, and it is only achieved through understanding. Therefore, we must seek after understanding as if it was gold or silver. Why? Because we tend only to do things we understand.

Children may be given principles to live by in the form of rules, but if they do not understand why the rule exists, they may never retain the principle in life. For example, we must first understand why reading the Bible is important if we are to pursue reading it. Understanding gives us the purpose to do it, and yet, understanding is not enough. It is only when we act on what we know and understand that wisdom is instituted.

3 Parts Wisdom (Spiritual)

It is a wonderful thing to read through the Bible in a year. However, when even one instance of spiritual knowledge is discovered, understood and applied to everyday life, it is a far greater accomplishment. The Bible is given to us, first to help us find salvation through Christ, then to teach God's principles and boundaries so that we may live a good, healthy, productive and abundant life here on earth.

In order to obtain this abundant life, we must extract from the Word the principles, values, morals, and faith to activate God's power. Power principles are essential to life. The power of faith alone can overcome obstacles, but principles can prevent obstacles from occurring in the first place. Therefore, we can see how both are critical for living a vibrant, successful and healthy life.

Spiritual well-being should not be measured by spiritual gifts or even by spiritual fruits, but rather, it should be measured by the integrity of our hearts. Does your heart desire to do right? Does your heart desire to please God? Does your heart feel sensitivity to the things of God? Does your heart care about others as much as you care about yourself?

Spiritual maturity is measured by your heart's condition, which in turn, is determined by the relationship you have with God, with others, and with yourself. Our heart believes circumstances can be changed by faith and that fate is controlled by the decisions we make according to God's Word. These beliefs are developed in the heart only by hearing, meditating, and acting on the Word of God. At the end of this book there is a list of scripture verses that you can confess every day. As you do so it will increase your level of faith and improve every area of your life, including physical health.

3 Parts Wisdom (Emotional)

Emotional well-being is reliant upon ultimate trust in God and the knowledge that He is good and has good in store for us. Some would say emotions are neither good nor bad, but just something we feel. This is not a true statement. There is good anger and bad anger; there is good love and love that is harmful; there is right sadness and wrong sadness, just to name a few. Most emotions can be expressed the wrong way and for wrong reasons. For example, God wants his children to be happy, but when we lose a loved one, we experience grief. This grief is okay as long as we emerge from it emotionally stronger than before.

Emotions are triggered by thoughts and thoughts, in turn, affect the heart. The heart affects actions because we do what we believe is appropriate. Therefore we must determine and control our thoughts and send to the heart the right signals so we have the correct behavior operating in our lives. If we control our thoughts and think on those things that are excellent, pure, honest, and praiseworthy, we will have a better system of checks and balances for our emotions. Take your thoughts captive; don't let your thoughts captivate you. You must become the captain of your ship. You may not be able to change the direction of the wind, but you can set your sails.

The Bible says, as a man thinks, so is he (Proverbs 23:7). In this scripture, the contextual meaning of "think" is "gate-keeper" or "custodian of the door." This means we have control of what we allow to make its way to our hearts, and thus affect our behavior. The mind decides what we believe by what is stored up in the heart. This in turn affects our gate-keeping job. Very little information is required to form a new belief, but it takes a great deal of information to change an old belief. It is equally difficult to change or adjust our actions, because we will always do what we believe.

3 Parts Wisdom (Physical)

Many things affect spiritual growth. Emotions, will and mind are all contributing factors. Further, our physical health affects both spiritual and emotional well-being. If we are physically sick, we do not feel like reading the Word, going to church or meditating on the Word. Therefore, we attain little spiritual growth. If we are physically sick, joy is difficult to experience. We take medication that slows down our thought processes, making it more difficult to think good thoughts. Thus, our emotions are affected. No amount of intelligence, money, relationships, notoriety, abilities, spirituality or psychology can do to our whole well-being what sickness can. Our health is critical.

How can we attain health or total well-being? Faith for health comes from consistently hearing the Word concerning health. This will produce health and healing if we eat right, sleep right and avoid harmful substances. We can follow God's principles and avoid needing a miracle for healing of sick bodies, but since we are human, we do not always live by these principles. Faith for health is important to spiritual and physical well-being.

Emotional well-being also has an effect on our physical health. Worry, stress, depression, fear, negative attitudes or any of these negative combinations can restrict blood flow and keep organs and cells in poor health. So physical, spiritual, and emotional well-being are all interconnected. All three must be developed and strengthened throughout life. We must grow in faith, in and through the Word of God. We must grow emotionally, in the fruits of the Spirit and develop the principles of God's Word. At the same time, we must take care of the temple God has given to us. Our goal is to be spirit men of power, emotional men of principles, and healthy men of strength so that we can act as complete bright lights and flavored salt and impact the world for Christ.

The Triune of Health

Physical
> Chiropractic
> Exercise
> Rest
> Breathe
> Massage

Chemical
> Eat raw, fresh, organic foods
> Drink water (distilled)
> Use whole food vitamins, minerals, and herbal
>   supplements
> Eliminate pharmaceutical and over-the-counter
>   drug use
> Remove internal and external poisons
> Cleanse colon, liver, kidney and cells
>   (with Doctor's consent)

Emotional
> Recite healing scriptures
> Positive, happy attitude
> Control, reduce negative stress
> Health affirmations
> Get outside. Stop and smell the roses

Chiropractic

The power that made the body heals the body. That power is housed in the nervous system. No cell, tissue, organ or system in your body can function or heal normally without constant direct communication from the brain through the spinal cord and nerves. Misaligned or subluxated vertebrae in the spinal column interfere and disrupt this communication, resulting in malfunctioning, diseased, and painful tissues. Chiropractic adjustments correct and restore misaligned vertebrae back to their normal position, not only restoring the proper nerve signals, but improving overall body posture, structure, and function. Minimum treatments of one a week to one per month are recommended.

Exercise

Daily exercise, including cardio, flexibility and strength are vital for overall fitness and function. Regular exercise will promote better circulation, coordination, mental wellness, chemical regulation, bone generation, nervous system and sleep patterns. Resistance exercise should be performed for the whole body 2-3 times per week. Cardiovascular should be done on an alternating schedule at the same frequency.

Rest

Sleep 6-8 hours per night. Get downtime between stressful activities and nap when you can. Repair and regeneration are essential parts of healing cycles. Ignore them at your peril.

Breathe

Deep breathing not only oxygenates your blood and tissues, the action itself is a key component in your body's complex energy management and healing system. Take ten deep breaths every morning—outside. Breathe in through your nose and out through your mouth, nice and slow.

Massage

Swedish, deep tissue and myofascial release are just a few types of massage. Each different application can help a variety of neuromuscular skeletal conditions from chronic muscle spasms and adhesions to fibromyalgia. Regular massage helps promote muscle tone, blood flow, and lymphatic drainage. It also helps the release of toxins and food poisons. Whether to promote healing to injured soft tissue or just to help relax, there is no substitute for a healing touch.

Health Potential

Health is something you are given at birth and it should be maintained throughout your lifetime. Unfortunately, we are never taught what we need for health and what specifically needs to be maintained.

We are all born with a genetic health potential. If we understand what can interfere with that potential, we can avoid such interferences and keep it at its highest level. When we buy a brand new car, we get a manual to maintain it. This tells us how to make the car last the longest possible time and run at its optimum potential with minimal problems. Yet, when children are born there is no manual in the "glove compartment" to know when to "change the oil," "rotate the tires" and get "tuned up." In other words, we are not taught what to maintain or how to maintain it. To understand how to obtain our highest optimum health potential, we first have to know what the essentials of health are.

To understand the essentials of health we need to understand the essentials of life. Many things could come to mind in different categories such as physiological, psychological or social. However, in terms of basic physiological essentials for survival we can name four. What makes these essential is that if any of them were to stop, you would die. If any of them were interfered with, your health would not be at its optimum potential.

The essentials of life are:

Food

Water

Oxygen

Nerve Impulse

Food

Food is the fuel and building blocks for growth and reproduction of cells and tissues. It consists of proteins, fats, and carbohydrates. If any of these were to stop you would die.

Water

75% of your body is water. It is used in almost every body reaction. If you stop fluid intake, you die.

Oxygen

Oxygen is also used in almost every reaction of the body and is carried by the pulmonary (lungs) and circulatory (blood) systems. Interference with these systems could stop oxygen and result in death.

Nerve Impulse

Nerve impulse is the most commonly over-looked essential for life and health. Nerve impulse is an electrochemical charge transmitted by the brain through the nervous system to the body. It is the life force that keeps us alive and "charged." All body function is dependent on this life force or brain impulse. Cells must be electrically charged in order to vibrate and function. If your brain stopped generating these electrical impulses, you would die.

Health's Hidden Enemy

In order to enjoy sound health, the individual must maintain structural balance of the spinal column. Any imbalance in structure or function will result in lowered immunity to disease.

It is the stresses, strains, knocks, and bumps of living that sometimes create this imbalance. Just look around you—heads forward, slumped shoulders, hollow backs, protuberant bellies, and rotated hips.

You can be sure these people suffer from attendant health problems such as back, heart, stomach, liver, sinus trouble, headaches, sciatica and ear infections, just to name a few. They may suffer from any of the nearly 400 different diseases or conditions caused by structural or functional imbalance.

Misaligned vertebrae which create interference are called subluxations. A fall or injury may produce subluxations. They may result from stresses or strain, either physically, chemically, or emotionally, which may overload the nervous system's protective mechanism.

Nervous System

When the nerve impulses flow smoothly and unimpeded as nature intends, a person enjoys health and a feeling of well-being. But when there is interference in normal nerve function, there will be imbalance either physically, chemically or emotionally. The spinal column is intended to protect the spinal cord and the nerves leading from it.

Should there be any loss of structural integrity, curvature, motion, restrictions or distortions of the spine, this could result in imbalance called subluxation. This imbalance causes interference with normal nerve function. Structure relates to function. Function relates to structure.

Structure Dictates Function

If you seek health, look first to the spine!

Socrates

The doctor should look well to the spine, for many diseases have their origin in vertebral displacements.

Hippocrates

The doctor of the future will give no medicine, but interest patients in the care of the human frame.

Thomas Edison

Abnormal structure predisposes the human body systems to abnormal biomechanics, abnormal function and ultimately pathological disorders.

American Journal of Pain Management 1994

Posture affects and moderates every physiological function from breathing to hormonal production.

American Journal of Pain Management 1994

Nutrition

The following is a list of things we can do for our physical well-being to maximize our health potential. These things are necessary because not only are our soils depleted, but also the chemicals released in the air and sprayed on plants are also significantly affecting us today in a negative way.

The nutritional community tells us we are attacked by 250 million free radicals a day under normal living conditions in America. These free radicals, or pollutants, pervert cells and rob them of nutrition.

These pollutants are only stopped by antioxidants, but most of our diets sorely lack these antioxidants. Therefore, we suffer the ravages of cancer, heart disease, diabetes, arthritis, Alzheimer's, memory loss, excessive tiredness, and early aging.

Free radicals tear down and deplete our immune systems, which in their weakened state no longer can enhance and activate our hormone-producing organs. This depleted state causes low hormone levels that slow down our metabolism and further weaken our immune system.

God gave us an awesome immune system capable of defeating any virus, bacteria or disease on earth, but we must feed the system the way He instructs us to and keep it strong, instead of destroying its resistance to disease and casting away our health.

Consider the following recommended intakes of nutrients for improving your overall well-being. This is not a cure-all or an instant fix, but rather a long-term way of life. Consistency will pay off in the end. It is never too late to start but it takes time to see changes and to feel changes. I believe that if you stick to these guidelines and take the supplements for 90 days, you will feel and look younger than you do now.

Note that you should never drink grapefruit juice with vitamins of any sort. It will negate the effects of the vitamins.

ESSENTIAL CRITICAL NUTRIENTS

Vitamin A	1000-5000 IU
	(Found in fish, fish oils, omegas)
	Helps clean the arteries
Beta Carotene	2500-100,000 IU *antioxidant*
Thiamine (B_1)	100-250 mg
Riboflavin (B_2)	50-250 mg
Pantothenic acid (B_5)	60-1000 mg
Niacin (B_3)	50-250 mg
Pyridoxine (B_6)	25-250 mg pyridoxal 5-phosphate
Cobalamin (B_{12})	500-1000 mg
Biotin	200-2000 (mcg)
Folic acid	800-2000 (mcg)
Vitamin C	600-3000 mg (Ester-C) *antioxidant*
Vitamin D	200-1000 IU
	(10 min. of sun also good source)
Vitamin E	400-1000 IU (mixed tocopherol)
	antioxidant

ESSENTIAL MINERALS

Drink pure water, either distilled or at least 98% purified, but remember, you must replace minerals you would normally get from water. Don't drink tap water.

Calcium	1000-2000 mg
Magnesium	500-1000 mg
Potassium	100-400 mg
Manganese	5-15 mg
Iron	10-40 mg
Chromium	100-600 (mcg)
Selenium	100-600 (mcg)
Boron	1-3 mg
Iodine	100-225 (mcg)
Copper	1-3 mg
Zinc	15-50 mg
Molybdenum	75-250 (mcg)
Vanadium	25-100 (mcg)

ESSENTIAL FATTY ACIDS

Flaxseed oil, capsules preferred   2000-10,000 mg
(An omega 3 fatty acid)
Provides skin fullness & elasticity
Gamma linoleic acid   250-500 mg (from borage oil)
(An omega 6 fatty acid)
Provides skin fullness & elasticity
Coenzyme Q10   50-300 mg
Antioxidant, Cleanse arteries
Fish oil 2000 mg   omega 3 and 6 fatty acids
Helps prevent clogging of arteries
Alpha lipoic acid 25 mg daily

ANTIOXIDANTS

COQ10   30-100 mg daily, 30 at a time
Pycnogenol. (French pine bark)   25-50 mg daily
Vitamin C   up to 4000 mg
Beta Carotine   2500-10,000 IU daily
Beta Glucan 1, 3   10 mg daily
Alpha lipoic acid   25 mg daily

ESSENTIAL FOR GOOD SKIN

All the above plus
L-Carnitine   500-4000 mg
Ester-C   600-2000 mg
Omega-3 fish oils
L-Tyrosene
L-Taurine
DMAE Caps (Dimethylaminoethanol)
CLA Supreme

The Plan

Get your doctor's permission to start.

Get a commitment letter signed and dated (between spouses or a friend who promises to hold you accountable).

Three days are exceptions:
> Thanksgiving, Christmas, and New Year's.

What to Eat:
- Fresh vegetables (green color best—frozen is okay, but not preferred).
- Fresh fruit (separated from meals by 2 hours).
- Chicken, no skin.
- Fish: deep cold water preferred (tuna, canned in water).
- Beef, extra lean.
- Turkey, no skin.
- Whole milk, cream, eggs, real butter.
- Bread: whole wheat, spelt, or Ezekiel.
- Fresh berries (dark color best).
- All raw nuts (no peanuts), almonds best, 10 per day snack.
- Soup is okay, homemade preferred.
- Juice, not from concentrate (single seed juice for weight loss, multi seed juice for weight gain).

1 cup coffee permitted daily. Separate from
meals by 2 hours.

Almond butter.

Herbal teas (all that you desire).

Green tea, one or more full cups daily.

Cereals, all whole grain cereals.

Use olive oil for cooking.

Honey, Splenda, Stevia, for sweetening.

Mayo (light), mustard, ketchup (limited).

Fast:

One day per week (if you have no sugar problems—hypo or hyperglycemic) with a doctor's permission.

Stop eating at 3 p.m. and fast until 6 a.m. the
following morning. Fast three days to
cleanse.

Drink unfiltered apple juice and distilled water
all you want.

Barley green recommended for second or third
day.

Distilled water with one fresh squeezed lemon
added, drink all you can.

Coming off of a fast, eat a light supper, no red
meat.

Normal Diet:

Eat hearty breakfasts and lunches.

Sleep 8 hours per 24-hour cycle.

Exercise at least 20 minutes, 3 times per week
(walking/stretching exercises).

An aerobic weight workout according to age and health.

Drink only bottled water (no tap water), pure filtered.

Get an acid/alkaline saliva test kit and keep your body slightly on the alkaline side.

30 grams of fiber capsules, or powder mix okay.

Eat only complex carbs after 3 p.m., no meat protein after 3 p.m.

Go to bed on an empty stomach!

Eat none of the following for 90 days:

No white flour or its products (use soy flour for baking).

No canned food (except soups and tuna in water).

No smoking/No alcohol.

No white sugar or white sugar products.

No scavenger meats, processed meats, canned meats.

No soda, not even diet.

No peanut products.

No margarine.

No processed cereals, only whole grain.

No tap water or water that has not been filtered.

A Balanced Diet

An important consideration in a healthy diet is maintaining a proper pH (potential of Hydrogen) balance. You can measure the acidity and alkalinity of your body by purchasing litmus paper that takes a measurement from your saliva.

If your body is too acidic, you will be more prone to a variety of diseases. A virus, for example, thrives in an acid environment. The goal is to keep a proper balance between acid and alkali.

The pH range for a human body that is considered ideal is between 6.8 and 7.0. When your level drops below pH 6.8 you are on the acidic side, a condition called acidosis. Levels that are above pH 7.0 are considered to be alkaline, or a condition called alkalosis.

Your pH level is affected by the types of food that you eat. You should eat a diet of about 50 percent raw foods. For most people a basic rule of thumb is to eat 80 percent alkaline-forming foods and 20 percent acid-forming foods every day.

If you have acidosis, some recommended foods are apples, avocados, bananas, bilberries, blackberries, grapefruit, grapes, lemons, pears, pineapples, strawberries and all vegetables. Fresh fruits, especially citrus fruits, and vegetables are the best. Cooked and processed foods tend to make the body acidic, as do animal proteins, especially beef and pork.

To reduce acidosis you should avoid beans, cereals, crackers, eggs, flour products, grains, oily foods, macaroni and sugar.

Alkalosis, the condition of being too alkaline, is not nearly as common as acidosis, but to deal with it requires a diet of acid producing foods. Eat about 80 percent grains, beans, breads, brown rice, crackers, lentils, macaroni, nuts, soy sauce and whole-grain cereals. The rest of the diet should be fresh fruits, vegetables, fish, chicken, eggs and natural cheese.

Juicing

The fresh juices mentioned in this book are ideally juiced in your kitchen and consumed immediately. Juicing is beneficial because it takes little energy to digest juice, and your body is getting plenty of necessary elements from the juice. Fruits and vegetables that are free of pesticides (organically grown) will provide optimum nutrition.

To make your own juices, you must first obtain a juicer. There are several good juicers on the market in many different price ranges.

Fresh fruit and vegetable juice is an excellent way to get vitamins, minerals, enzymes, proteins, carbohydrates, and chlorophyll. Many fruits and vegetables can be juiced with the peel still on to insure that all of the vitamins and minerals go into the juice. Juices should not be stored, because they slowly lose their nutrients.

Juices can be placed into roughly three categories:

1. **Green juices or green drinks:** Green juices stimulate cells and rejuvenate the body. They also build red blood cells. Green juices made from sprouts contain chlorophyll, which heals and cleanses the body. "Green drinks" can also be made by adding chlorophyll, purchased at your natural foods store, to juice. Green juices are made from spinach, celery, cabbage, dandelion greens, alfalfa sprouts, and other similar vegetables.

2. **Vegetable juices:** Fresh vegetables are restorers and builders. They help remove excess protein, fat, and acid wastes from the body. Vegetable juices help build the immune system and guard against illness.

3. **Fruit juices:** Fruit juices are cleansers. One favorite is watermelon juice. The seeds, rind and fruit can be juiced. Most juicers extract the pulp and leave you with clean, delicious juice. Watermelon juice is an excellent cleanser. Apples are delicious when juiced, as are citrus fruits and berries. Fruit juices are wonderful combined, too.

Fruit juices are best taken in the morning. Vegetable juices are best taken in the afternoon.

What does Dr. Anderson juice?
Ingredients recommended are per person.

3 stalks of celery
3 stalks of bok choy
$^1/_2$ dozen baby carrots
3 stalks of collard greens
6 spears of asparagus
handful of cranberries

Drink immediately for full effect on an empty stomach, then eat the regular meal.

The Juice Fast

The practice of fasting is as old as humanity. It has been a part of religious practice in virtually every culture and religion that has ever existed. It is usually thought of in terms of a religious practice associated with prayer but it is increasingly becoming a part of a regular health regimen for many people. It has significance for both the spirit and the body and the effects are similar for both.

As a part of prayer, fasting is a way of humbling yourself before God. It is essentially a means of renouncing or cutting off the physical in order to enhance the spiritual. In fact, the Hebrew word in the Old Testament for "fast" essentially means "cover over," as in covering over your mouth. When you fast, there is a kind of cleansing that goes on that brings a greater focus to your spiritual life.

It isn't that fasting twists God's arm to get Him to do things. Rather, it is you that changes as your spiritual hearing becomes clearer and you focus more on His will, rather than your own.

Fasting involves cleansing your soul of the things that hinder your spiritual life. By taking your attention away from food, you can redirect it to the things of God.

Fasting For Health

The physical effects of fasting are very similar. They produce a cleansing effect on the body by cleaning out accumulated toxins. The process of digesting food uses a tremendous amount of your energy. Significant amounts of blood are directed toward the stomach and the focus of the body is on the digestive system until the food is dealt with. When you stop eating, all of that energy can be directed at something else, specifically, cleaning the toxins out.

Your body is forced to take in toxins from a variety of sources—the food you eat, the air you breath, the water you drink and even the water you bathe in. The body has three ways of dealing with unhealthy substances. First it tries to burn them by converting them to energy. Much of it is also eliminated through digestion along with other waste.

Those two methods rid the body of most toxins but some are simply stored in a safe place. Your body tucks them away in fat cells where they won't do any immediate harm to healthy cells. Your body tries to protect the good cells and make the toxins ineffective. Basically, what isn't eliminated is hidden.

The Problem With Dieting

When people diet, they shrink the fat cells but the toxins stored in them remain. When people start to eat again, the body replaces the fat and the weight comes right back. The key to successful weight loss, that is, to losing it and keeping it off, is ridding the body of toxins first and then the fat cells. Then you need to maintain the cleansing by a once a month fast of three days. Do this and you will never be fat again.

When you begin a fast, the body starts cleaning out those storage places by dumping the toxins into your bloodstream to be eliminated. It is not hunger that causes you to feel so bad during a fast. It is the toxins that are flooding your system that give you headaches and nausea. It is an indication that you are getting cleaned out.

Regular Fasting

Regular fasting is good for you both spiritually and physically. It allows your body to rest, your organs to get cleaned out, your liver and kidneys to be cleansed, your blood purified and your colon to be cleansed. It is not just a spiritual thing. Fasting is a benefit to your whole being.

But if you are going to fast, you need to do it right or you can hurt yourself. This program is simple but it takes self-control and self-discipline. If you complete this program, food will never rule you again. You will eat to live and not live to eat. It is wonderful to have control of your own life.

You should always consult a physician if you intend to fast, just to make sure there are no complications that might arise from specific conditions. For example, if you are hypoglycemic or hyperglycemic, fasting can be dangerous. Check with your doctor first and check your blood sugar levels before, during and after the fast.

Types of Fasts

There are a variety of different types of fasts. I recommend a juice fast as the safest and most beneficial way to fast. It will help you keep your energy levels up while fasting so that you can continue to function fairly normally.

Length of a Fast

It is important to determine ahead of time exactly how long you are going to fast. Don't leave it open ended. Without a definite goal in mind, you will probably not last very long.

A fast can be as short as one meal. The longest fast recorded in the Bible was forty days. Usually a fast of one to three days is sufficient to give good benefits.

If you have never fasted before, you probably shouldn't start out with a long fast. A meal or one day is a good way to begin. In biblical times, it was common for people in the early church to fast twice a week for part of a day. They fasted every Wednesday and Friday until 4:00 p.m.

A fast of three days will get rid of most of the toxins in your system. A five-day fast will start healing in your body. After ten days, your body will be pretty much cleansed and you will have dropped 5-10 pounds, depending on your metabolism. It is good to do a three-day fast once a month and a seven to ten-day fast once or twice a year.

Preparation for a Fast

Many people have a large last meal before starting a fast. You should prepare for the fast by changing your diet to get rid of some of the toxins before the fast. It will make it much easier when you do fast. It is best to eat raw foods for at least two days before beginning a fast. If you are planning to fast for longer than three days, you might consider eating raw foods for longer.

During the Fast

Most people do not drink nearly enough water on normal days and you should double your water intake during a fast. Drink distilled water only. You can add lemon juice to it. The lemon becomes alkaline in your blood stream and neutralizes the acidic toxins.

Use only pure juices without sweeteners or additives. Avoid orange or tomato juice. The best are fresh lemon juice or unfiltered apple juice. Others are cabbage, beet, carrot, celery, and grape juice. "Green drinks," which are made from green leafy vegetables, are also good.

Avoid drinks like tea, coffee and all soft drinks.

The 40-Day Juice Fast

Here is a simple 40 day fast that you can do. Stay continually in touch with your physician.

Day 1

Apple juice (unfiltered)
Distilled water
No food

Day 2

Diluted apple juice (50/50 with distilled water)

Day 3

Distilled water with fresh squeezed lemons

Days 4-7

Vegetable juice (fresh) morning and evening, made with:
celery — 3 stalks
carrot — 1 whole
bok choy —1 large stalk
cabbage — 1" slice
beet — $1/2$ with leaves
apple — 1 whole

Days 7-40

Same except add a whey protein shake with water
  or whole milk at least every other day.
High protein—Low Carb

Vitamins and Supplements
Vitamin C—3000 mg with juice
Vitamin E—400 IU with juice
Vitamin B—100 mg with juice
Beta Carotene—25,000 mg with juice
Alpha Lipoic Acid—200 mg with juice
Glutathione—100 mg with juice (sublingual best)
COQ10—30 mg
A mineral supplement with trace minerals
A multi vitamin, dissolvable (Test tablet over-
    night in water. If it doesn't dissolve, find
    one that does.)
Fiber—30 mg daily (powder)
PB8 Acidophulus—1 weekly

Drink only bottled water (at least 6 glasses per day, no
    tap water)
When traveling and unable to juice, try Green Power
    Juice, Barley Green or Green Drink, Super Greens
Bathe daily with a health bar of soap (no additions)
Scrub down with Soft Body (scrub external detox)
Bathe after swimming in chlorinated water

Exercise During a Juice Fast
    It will not hurt you to exercise during a fast, but
your energy levels will be reduced so you might want to
reduce the amount of exercise you engage in. Remember
that it is all right to rest. If the fast leaves you tired, just
lay down and rest. It will do your body good and it will
help you to get through the more difficult part of a fast.
Remember, you feel bad because your body is dumping

toxins into your blood stream. But that is good. They need to be cleaned out. Just rest whenever you can. You should probably plan a fast for days when you can rest, if possible, rather than while you are working.

Breaking a Fast

After the first day of a fast, your digestive system starts to shut down, since it isn't getting any food. A fast also cleans out the bacteria that are necessary to break food down. You should not shock your system by dumping a steak on top of it when it has been resting for several days. You could actually do great harm to yourself if you don't come off of a fast gradually.

As a general rule, you should take at least one day to come off of a fast for every three days that you have been on it. Do not begin with anything cooked, greasy or heavy. You should start with a raw salad or some fruit. Build up to normal meals over a period of time. There is no hurry. Also remember that your stomach contracts while you are fasting so you will not need large portions to fill you up.

Done properly, a fast is extremely beneficial, both spiritually and physically. It is wise to begin making it a regular part of your lifestyle. It will take some discipline but if you observe common sense in the way that you approach fasting and stick to it faithfully, you will experience greater health, more energy and honest weight loss.

Anti-Aging

Hormone levels naturally produced by our own bodies begin to decline as we age. While the most dramatic drop is seen between 45 and 50 in most people, the tapering-off process begins around the age of 35.

There are numerous reasons why hormone production declines, but perhaps the most obvious reason is that both the food we eat and the water we drink lack the minerals and nutrition we need. Because hormone levels affect our immune systems and the ability of our bodies to fight off disease, the lower hormone levels we have, the faster the aging process, and the more susceptible we become to sickness.

With the aid of your nutritional medical doctor, you can increase and regulate your hormones so that they return to the levels you had in your twenties, thus slowing aging, lessening the chances of disease, and quite possibly lengthening your life. Although I recommend a doctor to oversee and regulate your hormonal therapy, you can take some immediate steps.

For men, DHEA is a powerful fighter of aging. This hormone can be purchased at local health stores and has been shown to enhance immunity as well as reducing the risk of heart attacks, cancer, and diabetes. DHEA studies have shown improvement in physical and psychological health.

Women: 10-25 mg daily (Keto is a form of
           DHEA for women)
Men: 10-100 mg daily

Pregnenolone can also be purchased over the counter. This awesome hormone slows aging, enhances memory and intelligence, and also improves mood, boosts energy, and increases overall alertness and awareness.

BRAIN ENHANCERS

Phosphatidylchlorine	100 mg
Phosphatidylserine	100-300 mg
Acetyl L-Carnitine	500-3000 mg
Ginkgo biloba	25 mg

CLEANSERS

Fiber	25 grams daily (psyllium husks)

ANTI-AGING HERBS

Ginseng   25-75 mg
                 energy & sexual drive
Ginkgo   120-240 mg
                 clear mind & immune system
Garlic (Kyolic)   500-2000 mg
                 antioxidant cleans blood

ANTI-AGING HORMONES

DHEA	10-100 mg
Pregnenolone	25-200 mg
Melatonin	5-10 mg
Estrogen**	natural creams
Progesterone**	natural creams
Testosterone**	natural creams

Thyroid** (Not for everyone)
    (If you use thyroid it needs to be taken on
    an empty stomach, with nothing else, or it
    won't have any effect.)

L-Tyrosene	500 mg, 2x daily
ThyroStart	(Name Brand)
Kelp	200 mg

** All require a doctor's prescription and monitoring.

Anti-Aging, Youth Restoring Hormones In Detail

Melatonin is a hormone that is produced naturally by the pineal gland, which is located between your eyes and behind your nose. When darkness is sensed, melatonin is released into the body to produce drowsiness so the body rests well. The purpose of rest is to rebuild damaged areas as well as replace every cell in the body every seven years.

    Melatonin production slowly declines as we grow older, and seemingly, older people need less sleep. They tend to get up earlier and earlier. In fact, the opposite is true. As we age we need more sleep for repair, but because less melatonin is produced, we rest less, thus promoting aging.

Melatonin replacement is a good thing but too much can be a bad thing. A good measuring stick for trying melatonin is to take just enough so that you sleep 8 hours and wake up rested. Therefore, you can be assured that your body is getting its needed rest.

Try one gram of time-released melatonin at first. Then if more is needed, add one gram more until the proper amount is established. If you awake and yawn throughout the day, you have taken too much. Time-released is best.

Estrogen is produced naturally in a woman's body. As aging sets in at 35 to 40 years, the body produces less and less. Estrogen is prescribed by doctors and has been for years, but the problem is most prescriptions are synthetic. Synthetic estrogen can cause cancer. If you take Estrogen, make sure it is natural. Estrogen will help chemically balance your body's hormones and minimize mood swings caused by menopause or PMS.

Progesterone declines sharply after menopause. Low or lacking progesterone is the cause of osteoporosis and it speeds aging. Natural progesterone therapy adjusted by a physician can somewhat reverse osteoporosis or stop it.

Testosterone is a powerful male hormone. It controls the sex drive, builds muscle mass and promotes strength and energy. You should check your levels with a physician every three months. Testosterone levels peak in men between 16 and 21 years of age and begin to decline for the rest of life. By the age of 45-50, some men sense a decline of interest in sex and loss of energy levels. Fat replaces muscles. These controlling physical effects and negative thinking processes set men up for mid life crisis. As the testosterone shortage decreases his interest in sex, a man tends to blame it on his wife, her attractiveness, or on life in general. Men are tempted to relive their youth, to find that strong sexuality they remember.

Men, the answer is not someone else or something else; it is testosterone hormone therapy. The key is to rebuild your testosterone level back to what it was when you were 30. Under a doctor's care, you will see your fat turn back to muscle (exercise is required in conjunction), and you will experience youthful energy and renewed sexual interest.

Women, if you are experiencing a lack of sexual interest, it may be a result of low testosterone. Yes, women also must maintain a small amount of this hormone in order to have the energy and desire for sexual intimacy. In addition, testosterone will also lower the risk of heart attack and slow the aging process drastically.

The **thyroid hormone** is perhaps the most neglected, but also most depleted hormone of all. A significant number of people in the world suffer from thyroid problems. The thyroid hormone, which is produced by the thyroid gland at the base of the throat, diminishes as we grow old. This low thyroid production affects your immune system and its ability to ward off diseases. Weight gain, anemia, heart disease and irregular heart rates are all related to low thyroid production.

To test your thyroid, shake down a mercury thermometer before bed. Upon waking, and before any movement, place the thermometer under your arm for ten minutes. If the reading is under 97.2, you probably have a slow thyroid and a doctor's prescription should be sought to enhance production by taking natural thyroid.

Finally, do not let your brain age too quickly. There are things called **neuron nutrients**, and by using them you can improve your memory, raise your IQ and slow the aging of your mind.

The two most potent brain nutrients are **Ginkgo Biloba** and the hormone **pregnenolone**. Also important is **Acetyl L-Carnitine (ALC)** which sharpens memory, alertness and learning recall.

Phosphatidylserine (PS) belongs to a special category of fat-soluble substances called phospholipids, which are essential components of cell membranes. PS is found in high concentrations in the brain and may help preserve, or even improve, some aspects of mental functioning, memory, alertness and brain energy when supplements are taken.

The program laid out for taking all of the nutrients we have discussed will have limited effects and benefits based on the following:

1. Quality of Products

It is essential that quality products be purchased from a reputable health food store. There are many great products available today and many new ones coming out. Don't trust just anyone; check it out for yourself.

2. Consistency of Use

Consistency is vital. Good health is not something to try. It is a way of life. When you start, do not stop. Be consistent and persistent! In some cases, it may take a year to see noticeable benefits, but consistency is essential to reap the greatest long term benefits.

3. Ability to be Absorbed into the Body

Proper absorption of nutrients into the body is dependent on the condition of the colon; therefore a clean, healthy colon is essential for overcoming sickness and disease and must not be neglected.

Most Americans do not eat enough fiber (30 grams per day) to keep the colon clean. In addition, we eat simple carbohydrates, white sugar, and white flour. These refined foods create sludge in the colon and coat it, killing healthy bacteria and slowing absorption of nutrients into the blood. The colon is capable of carrying 35 to 40 pounds of sludge. This sludge slows absorption and tells the body to eat more and bigger meals to get enough food.

This cycle causes a craving for more and more sugar, and more weight gain. Clean the colon, lose weight, feel better, have more energy, and be healthy. Colon cleansing can be done by a licensed physician and is very beneficial. In order to keep and maintain healthy bacteria in your clean colon, be sure to eat plenty of fiber and supplement with fiber tablets and the friendly bacteria acidophilus and bifidus (mother's milk) daily.

All of the things I have discussed are essential to building a healthy body—the ultimate defense system. I am told that 200 million free radicals attack the body every day (by infiltration from sources such as bad food, the air we breathe, and skin contact). You must take enough antioxidants and nutrients to fortify the immune system while drinking enough clean, healthy water to flush out all the junk. A strong immune system can defeat every disease, virus, and bacteria on earth. Your immune system will keep you healthy if you keep it healthy.

40+ Generation

Flexibility Training and Aerobic Fitness
for the 40+ Generation
by Colman R. Foster

O ur body is the temple of our living God, and His almighty Spirit lives in us. Paul brings this concept out in 1 Corinthians 3:16. Paul also states in 1 Corinthians 6:19, "You are not our own." Yes, our body does belong to our Father God.

With this in mind, I believe it is incumbent on a person who has a relationship with Jesus to work on a physical fitness program. Physical fitness in the development of the body to a state of condition which promotes the performance of a given amount of physical work, when desired, with a minimum amount of physical effort.

As a physical educator and coach for over thirty years, I taught the value of aerobic fitness and flexibility to my students. I believe to stay fit in life, we need to eat right and be involved in a physical fitness program. Apart from the physical fitness program, there should be concentration on aerobic fitness and flexibility training.

Flexibility is the capacity of bending and stretching. In developing flexibility, the goal should be to develop a state of elasticity to prevent muscle injury. In my coaching experiences, I found three types of muscle injuries—the muscle strain, the muscle pull and the torn muscle. These injuries can be prevented by taking the necessary time to stretch prior to the physical workout.

Again, stretching creates limberness and elasticity of the muscles that minimizes the chance of muscle problems while doing physical activities. The goal in aerobic fitness is to develop an average amount of oxygen consumption, as measured by the 12 minute field test created by Dr. Kenneth Cooper.

As a sixty-four year old person, I have modified this test to fit my needs. I will tell you why as we go along. This test requires a person to complete as many laps as possible on a 400 meter track in a 12 minute time period. One can walk or run to complete the distance.

The following is my modification of the 12 minute field test:

> 1-2 laps = poor oxygen consumption.
> 3-4 laps = average consumption.
> 5-6 laps = good oxygen consumption.

This test determines the amount of oxygen intake or aerobic capacity that is measured in milliliters of oxygen per kilogram per minute.

Dr. Kenneth Cooper, in his two books, *Aerobics* and *New Aerobics*, examines the importance of aerobics on a person's life-style. A person's capacity, as discussed by Cooper, is the capacity to take in oxygen. He states that "this is important because aerobic fitness produces the training effect." The training effect produces the following:

1. It strengthens the muscles or respiration and tends to reduce the resistance to air flow.

2. It improves the strength and pumping efficiency of the heart.

3. It tones up the muscles throughout the body, therefore improving general circulation.

4. It causes an increase in the total amount of blood circulating in the body and increases the number of red blood cells.

In the book *Physiology of Exercise*, by Laurence Morehouse, the author states, "Maximal oxygen intake during strenuous exercise or exertion declines slowly with advancing age. A subject who is able to use 4 liters of oxygen per minute at the age of twenty years will probably be able to use not more than 3 liters per minute at age fifty." This information is why I modified Dr. Cooper's 12 minute test.

As a person under fifty, I was able to meet the criteria in Dr. Cooper's 12 minute test. His test has the average performance at 5 laps; 6 laps represents a good performance. I used myself as a test study and I found my 4 lap performance was equal to the 5 lap performance of years gone by. I still do the same workouts I did when I completed the 5 laps in 12 minutes.

Needless to say that physical degeneration takes place with the aging process, but we can slow this process down by exercise. Remember that all exercises must be done slowly and according to what can be done. Exercise and the fitness process is not a contest.

For the training effect to take place, a person must get their pulse rate up to 120 beats per minute. I found the best way for a person to take their own pulse is with the fingers at the carotid artery. Place the fingers at about 3 inches below the left or right ear lobe at the throat. The best way to have the pulse rate go up is to run, but there are optional methods for the desired result. One can bicycle, walk fast, swim or use low impact exercise machines, to mention some options to running.

Terminology:

1. Repetition: (REP) An execution of an exercise from a starting position, back to a starting position.

2. Set: Execution of an exercise for a given number of repetitions. One set may consist of anywhere from 3-20 repetitions.

An exercise may be performed at any number from 2-4 sets (rest between sets is recommended).

Calisthenics or Warm-Up:

Before starting the physical fitness program, one needs to get a doctor's okay for the proposed program. Before doing the actual aerobic exercise, it is necessary to warm up with a stretching routine.

Calisthenics or Cals, which are generally referred to as warm-up exercises, have a definite purpose in a physical fitness program. They are exercises that are used as a warm-up or preliminary to more strenuous activity. To obtain this purpose they must be carried out energetically and with complete dedication. It has been found that muscles are more effective after the initial warm-up and are less susceptible to injury.

Exercise Routine

The following routine is what I directed with my physical education classes and athletic teams.

Warm-up and Stretching Exercises:

10-20 repetitions of each exercise should be done before every aerobic fitness work-out.

Jumping Jacks or Jumping Rope

Start the warm-up period with five minutes of jumping jacks or jump rope. This activity increases body temperature and speeds up circulation along with aiding coordination and agility.

Bend and Reach

From a standing position with feet spread, thrust the arms through the legs. Do this in a three count motion. Do not bounce. Bouncing causes quick contractions and could cause a muscle strain. On the fourth count, come to the starting position. (3-5 sets)

Side Bend

From the previous position, lean to the left (stretching the inside of the left leg) for 10-15 counts. Repeat leaning on the right. (Remember, do not bounce.)

Bottoms Up

Starting with the feet spread 20 inches apart, place fingers on the ground and hold for 2 counts on a full stretch, if possible. Return to the starting position and repeat.

Leg Cross Over

Stand with legs straight. Put the right leg over the left leg and bend slowly without any bounce. Repeat with the left leg over the right leg. (10-20 counts)

Toe Raisers

Stand flat footed and rise to tip toes. This activity stretches the lower legs. (10-13 reps, three sets)

Wall Lean

Stand and lean into a wall or a solid object with the left knee and left leg forward and the right leg back. Place the right heel downward to the floor. Repeat the process with the right leg. (10-20 counts per leg)

Hip Pull

Sit down and bring the right leg over the extended left leg as fast as possible to the left hip and pull gently on the right knee. This activity stretches the upper leg and buttocks area. Repeat the process with the other leg. (10-15 counts)

Backward Lean

Sit on the knees with the knees on the floor and lean slowly backwards to stretch the quads. (Hold for 10 counts)

Upper Body Stretch

Stand erect with hands together above the head and lean to the right and lean to the left. (10-15 counts on each side)

After stretching, start the aerobic portion of the workout using the desired method of choice. The main consideration a person must realize is one must do the activity a minimum of twelve minutes after the heart rate is 120 beats per minute. The longer one goes after 12 minutes, the more aerobic development takes place. If the person is tired at the point of 120 beats per minute, stop and resume when able to continue.

Do not exceed thirty minutes to start. Do not overdo the activity; listen to your body. What is the body saying? Is there abnormal breathing or is there abnormal feelings in the muscles? If so, STOP. The heart rate measures the desired amount of the activity.

When starting the exercise program, only do what is comfortable. Do not start breathing hard or hyper-ventilating. Start easy and rest as the pulse rate dictates. Check the pulse rate frequently.

Our fitness program should produce elasticity of the muscles to prevent muscle injury and develop an aerobic capacity to breathe without laboring in a desired activity.

Dr. Anderson's
18 Minute Exercise Program

Much research has been done on exercise to maintain health and conditioning. There is a minimum of exercise necessary—2 miles of walking. Purchase a pedometer to measure your normal motion daily. You might be surprised.

First of all, always park far from work, the store, the shops and anywhere else that you go. Make yourself walk. Even if it is only a short distance, any walking is better than no walking. Walk briskly when you walk. Avoid easy walking or waddling. My daily walking exceeds three miles—every day, seven days a week.

In addition to walking, my three-day-a-week program is as follows:

6 minutes on a stairstepper, climbing 50 stories.

Move quickly to 2 minutes at 4.0 on a treadmill.

Move to bench press (chest, shoulder, triceps)
    set of 12 light, set of 12 heavy.

Pull downs (back, lats, biceps, neck)
    12 light, 12 heavy
    hands apart on first 12
    hands close on second 12

12 butterflies with free weight
25 lbs. (shoulders and chest)

15 curls
Stationary arms, each with 25 lbs.

5 curls with 35 lbs.

Shower

Total time: 18 minutes

The Power of Confession

The confession of our mouths is as important as anything we do for our health. When we learn to confess the Word, we will find our attitudes changing, our emotional outlook becoming better and our physical health improving.

Below are confessions that are based on God's promises in the Bible. These words tell us what God desires for your health. If you begin every day speaking them out loud, it will produce life, health and stability in you, and many of the nutritional and diet elements that you have struggled with will become easy.

I speak the truth of the Word of God in love and I grow up into the Lord Jesus Christ in all things. (Ephesians 4:15)

No man shall take me out of my Father's hand for I have eternal life. (John 10:29)

I let the peace of God rule in my heart and I refuse to worry about anything. (Colossians 3:15)

I will not let the Word of God depart from before my eyes for it is life to me; for I have found it and it is health and healing to all my flesh. (Proverbs 4:21-22)

God is on my side. God is in me now. Who can be against me? He has given to me all things that pertain to life and godliness. Therefore I am a partaker of His divine nature. (2 Corinthians 6:16; John 10:10; 2 Peter 1:3-4; Romans 8:31)

Jesus gave me the authority to use His name. And that which I bind on earth is bound in heaven. And that which I loose on earth is loosed in heaven. Therefore, in the name of Jesus Christ, I bind the principalities, the powers, the rulers of the darkness of this world. I bind and cast down spiritual wickedness in high places and render them harmless and ineffective against me in the name of Jesus. (Matthew 16:19; John 16:23-24; Ephesians 6:12)

I am complete in Him who is the head of all principalities and powers. For I am His work-manship, created in Christ Jesus unto good works which God has before ordained that I should walk therein. (Colossians 2:10; Ephesians 2:10)

For Appetite Control

In the name of Jesus, I speak to my body and command my thoughts about food to line up with good nutrition. I bind any spirit of lust, sugar, fat, pork, blood, too much meat, junk food and all other unhealthy foods.

I speak to my body and command my metabolism to become perfectly normal. Digestive organs, I command you to work in the name of Jesus.

I speak to my appetite and command it to be healed at the normal limits, in the name of Jesus. I will no longer experience a ferocious appetite, or be tempted to go on eating binges.

I say, appetite, you will learn to love pleasant bread and you will eat it willingly, without murmuring, for the Glory of God and the sake of the Kingdom, in the name of Jesus. Amen. (Romans 12:1; 1 Corinthians 6:19-20)

For God is at work within me, helping me to obey Him, and then helping me to do what He wants. (Philippians 2:13)

The Lord will perfect that which concerns me. (Psalm 138:8)

Jesus is made unto me wisdom, righteousness, sanctification and redemption. Therefore I confess I have the wisdom of God, and I am the righteousness of God in Christ Jesus. (1 Corinthians 1:30; 2 Corinthians 5:21)

I am filled with knowledge of the Lord's will in all wisdom and spiritual understanding. (Colossians 1:9)

I am a new creation in Christ, I am His workman-
ship created in Christ Jesus. Therefore, I have the
mind of Christ and the wisdom of God is formed
within me. (2 Corinthians 5:17; Ephesians 2:10;
1 Corinthians 2:16)

I receive the Spirit of wisdom and revelation
in the knowledge of Him, the eyes of my understanding being enlightened. And I am not
conformed to this world, but I am transformed
by the renewing of my mind. My mind is renewed by the Word of God. (Ephesians 1:17-18;
Romans 12:2)

Overweight

I don't desire to eat so much that I become overweight. I present my body to God. My body
is the temple of the Holy Ghost which dwells
in me. I am not my own, I am bought with a
price, therefore, in the name of Jesus, I refuse
to overeat. Body, settle down, in the name of
Jesus, conform to the Word of God. I mortify
the desires of this body and command it to come
into line with the Word of God. (Romans 12:1;
1 Corinthians 6:19)

Healthy Bones and Marrow

Father, I make a demand on my bones to produce
perfect marrow. I make a demand on the marrow

to produce pure blood that will ward off sickness and disease. My bones refuse any offense of the curse. (Proverbs 16:24)

Immune System

My immune system grows stronger day by day. I speak life to my immune system. I forbid confusion in my immune system. The same Spirit that raised Christ from the dead dwells in me and quickens my immune system with the life and wisdom of God, which guard the life and health of my body. (Romans 8:2, 11)

Heart and Blood

Thank you, Father, that I have a strong heart. My heart beats with the rhythm of life. My blood flows to every cell of my body, restoring life and health abundantly. (Proverbs 12:14; 14:30)

My blood pressure is 120 over 80. The life of God flows in my blood and cleanses my arteries of all matter that does not pertain to life. (Mark 11:23)

My heart beat is normal. My heart beats with the rhythm of life, carrying the life of God throughout my body, restoring life and health abundantly. (Romans 8:1; Ephesians 2:22)

I have a strong heart. Every heartbeat floods my body with life and cleanses me of disease and pain. (Exodus 23:25; Mark 11:23)

I command my blood cells to destroy every disease germ and virus that tries to inhabit my body. I command every cell of my body to be normal in Jesus' name. (Romans 5:17; Luke 17:6)

Every cell that does not promote life and health in my body is cut off from its life source. My immune system will not allow tumorous growths to live in my body in Jesus' name. (Luke 17:6; Mark 11:23)

I am redeemed from the curse of the law and my heart beats with the rhythm of life. The Spirit and life of God's Word flows in me, cleansing my blood of every disease and impurity. (Galatians 3:13; Proverbs 4:20-23)

Arteries and Cells

In Jesus' name, my arteries will not shrink or become clogged. Arteries, you are clean, elastic and function as God created you to function. (Luke 17:6; Mark 11:23; Isaiah 55:11)

The law of the Spirit of Life in Christ Jesus has made me free from the law of sin and death; therefore, I will not allow sin, sickness or death to lord over me. (Romans 6:13-14; 8:2)

The same Spirit that raised Jesus from the dead dwells in me, permeating His life through my veins, sending healing throughout my body. (Romans 8:11)

In Jesus' name I forbid my body to be deceived in any manner. Body, you will not be deceived by any virus or disease germs. Neither will you work against life and health in any way. Every cell of my body supports life and health. (Matthew 12:25, 35)

Enforcing Life

Body, I speak the Word of faith to you. I demand that every internal organ perform a perfect work, for you are the temple of the Holy Ghost; therefore, I charge you in the name of the Lord Jesus Christ and by the authority of His Holy Word to be healed and made whole in Jesus' Name. (Proverbs 12:18; 1 Corinthians 3:16)

Father, I resist the enemy in every form that he comes against me. I require my body to be strong and healthy, and I enforce it with your Word. I reject the curse, and I enforce life in this body. (James 4:7)

You have forgiven all my iniquities; you have healed all my diseases; you have redeemed my life from destruction; you have satisfied my

mouth with good things so that my youth is renewed as the eagles. (Psalm 103:2-5)

I will not die but live and declare the works of
God. (Psalms 118:17)

Lord, you have blessed my food and water and
have taken sickness away from me. Therefore,
I will fulfill the number of my days in health.
(Exodus 23:25-26)

God's Daily Medicine

Jesus is the Lord of my life. Sickness and disease
have no power over me. I am forgiven and free
from sin and guilt. I am dead to sin and alive to
righteousness. (Colossians 1:21, 22)

I am free from unforgiveness and strife. I forgive
others as Christ has forgiven me, for the love
of God is shed abroad in my heart by the Holy
Ghost. (Matthew 6:12; Romans 5:5)

You have given me abundant life. I receive that
life through your Word and it flows in every
organ of my body, bringing healing and health.
(John 6:63; 10:10)

Heavenly Father, I attend to your Word. I incline
my ears to your sayings. I will not let them depart from my eyes. I keep them in the midst of

my heart, for they are life and healing to all my flesh. (Proverbs 4:20-22)

As God was with Moses, so is He with me. My eyes are not dim; neither are my natural forces abated. Blessed are my eyes for they see and my ears hear. (Deuteronomy 34:7)

No evil will befall me, neither shall any plague come near my dwelling. For you have given your angels charge over me. They keep me in all my ways. In my pathway is life, healing and health. (Psalm 91:10-11; Proverbs 12:28)

To Defeat Worry and Fear

I am the body of Christ and Satan has no power over me. For I overcome evil with good. (1 Corinthians 12:27; Romans 12:21)

I am of God and have overcome (Satan). For greater is He that is in me than he that is in the world. (1 John 4:4)

I will fear no evil for you are with me, Lord. Your Word and your Spirit comfort me. (Psalm 23:4)

I am far from oppression, and fear does not come near me. (Isaiah 54:14)

No weapons formed against me will prosper, for my righteousness is of the Lord. But whatever I do will prosper for I'm like a tree planted by the rivers of water. (Isaiah 54:17; Psalm 1:3; Jeremiah 17:8)

I am delivered from the evils of this present world, for it is the will of God. (Galatians 1:4)

I am a doer of the Word of God and am blessed in my deeds. I am happy in those things which I do because I am a doer of the Word of God. (James 1:22)

I take the shield of faith and I quench every fiery dart that the wicked one brings against me. (Ephesians 6:16)

I am an overcomer and I overcome by the blood of the lamb and the word of my testimony. (Revelation 12:11)

I am submitted to God, and the devil flees from me because I resist him in the name of Jesus. (James 4:7)

The Word of God is forever settled in heaven. Therefore, I establish His Word upon this earth. (Psalm 119:89)

Great is the peace of my children for they are taught of the Lord. (Isaiah 54:13)

The confessions on the preceding pages are based on scripture and personalized so that you can get a greater grasp of the promises of God for you concerning your health and well being. Below are some direct quotes from the Word of God about health. Learn them, speak them and make them a part of your daily life, as much as you would food, for they are life and health.

> Pleasant words are like a honeycomb,
> Sweetness to the soul and health to the bones.
> (Proverbs 16:24)

So you shall serve the LORD your God and He will bless your bread and your water. And I will take sickness away from the midst of you. (Exodus 23:25)

> My son, give attention to my words;
> Incline your ear to my sayings.
> Do not let them depart from your eyes;
> Keep them in the midst of your heart;
> For they are life to those who find them,
> And health to all their flesh.
> Keep your heart with all diligence,
> For out of it spring the issues of life.
> (Proverbs 4:20-23)

> He sent His word and healed them,
> And delivered them from their destructions.
> (Psalm 107:20)

My son, do not forget my law,
But let your heart keep my commands;
For length of days and long life
And peace they will add to you.
(Proverbs 3:1-2)

Bless the LORD, O my soul;
And forget not all His benefits:
Who forgives all your iniquities,
Who heals all your diseases,
Who redeems your life from destruction,
Who crowns you with lovingkindness and
    tender mercies,
Who satisfies your mouth with good things,
So that your youth is renewed like the eagle's.
(Psalm 103:2-5)

Moses was one hundred and twenty years old
when he died. His eyes were not dim nor his
natural vigor diminished. (Deuteronomy 34:7)

In righteousness you shall be established;
You shall be far from oppression, for you
    shall not fear.
And from terror, for it shall not come near you.
(Isaiah 54:14)

For I am the LORD who heals you. (Exodus 15:26)

A merry heart does good, like medicine.
(Proverbs 17:22)

The 90 Day Challenge

by Tammy Zubeck and Heather Murray

(This section was written by two winners of the 90 Day Challenge held in early 2004. They wanted to help others realize that eating the 90 Day way is not as difficult or as expensive as people might think. There is some initial work as you retrain yourself and work healthy eating into your schedule, but the payoff is worth it!)

Now that you've got the information of what to eat and why to eat it, you need to know how and where to get started. There are many stores that specialize in organic foods and most grocery stores carry many of the things that you need. You will have to check the yellow pages or get online to find the stores in your area. Finding healthy, whole, organic foods is not difficult, nor is it as expensive as one may think. Besides, now that you won't be spending money on soda, packaged dinners, and junk food, you'll probably find your grocery bill staying around the same amount as before, and it might even be lower.

When we first started the 90 Day program, we tried a new store every week. And we went without the kids so we could take the time to read labels! Reading labels is the key to good grocery shopping. Once you find your niche and you get used to your store, you can bring the kids.

The caveat is that you can't just go to these stores and buy everything because they are "health food" stores. You still have to read the labels. Remember to think "Fresh." You want fresh fruits, fresh vegetables, fresh meats—no processed, packaged, frozen, or canned. In general, you are looking for ingredients you can pronounce. You don't necessarily have to buy everything organic, but they are grown to higher standards. Try looking for some cereals, granolas, baking ingredients, beans, rice, and pastas in the bulk food section. You can buy just enough to taste and be sure you like it before buying more. Here is what you should look for when shopping for different items:

Breads – whole grains, not enriched, sweetened with honey okay.

Cereals – Kashi, granola

Cereal bars – fruit, whole grains, sweetened with honey

Crackers – Kashi, whole wheat sweetened with honey

Eggs – from grain-fed, free-range chicken (no antibiotics), high in DHA, Omega-3's

Juices – not from concentrate

Mayonnaise – canola oil, eggs, no sugar

Meats –lean ground beef (no growth hormone); grain-fed, free-range chicken (no antibiotics); fresh chicken or turkey sausage (no nitrates); fish

Olive oil – extra virgin cold expeller pressed

Pasta – durum semolina wheat, not enriched

Salsa – if you can't make your own, at least look
    for organic vegetables and no sugar
Tortillas – whole grain, no partially hydroge-
    nated oils
Tortilla Chips – white, yellow, or blue corn; cano-
    la, sunflower, or safflower oil, not partially
    hydrogenated; sea salt; lime (optional)

You can take almost any recipe you have and substitute healthier ingredients. Following are a few examples of ones that we have done. There are many other recipes available. You have only to take the time to look for them. The only thing we haven't been able to successfully locate is a substitute for cream soups in a lot of the casserole recipes. So we've inserted some busy mom tips for those of you who need those time-saving recipes that the casseroles used to afford you.

Another tip: Don't be afraid to mix and match or be creative with the eating needs of your own family. As you continue to familiarize yourself with this whole new concept of eating you will find that your family will have favorites and you will come to know what works and does not work for you and your family.

Look for opportunities to organize your shopping and cooking tactics and keep those shelves stocked. We buy at least two of everything so we're not constantly running to the store. When we use one of the two items stocked, we then place that item on our grocery list and replace it on the next run. Constantly have your shelves stocked and you'll be at ease with your whole shopping/cooking experience. Remember, God WILL supply all your needs!

Breakfast:

Eggs and Hash Browns

Cook two eggs any style; try using canola, safflower, sunflower, or olive oil instead of butter. Shred your own potatoes and freeze them so they are ready ahead of time, or you can find frozen organic hash browns at some stores. Some people only need the protein in the morning, while others find that they need the protein and carbs to feel full through the morning.

Almond Butter and Honey Sandwich
On Whole Wheat Bread

A good protein/carb balanced breakfast. Follow up with fruit a couple hours later.

Fruit Smoothie With Protein Powder

In a blender, combine one cup of orange juice or papaya nectar, half a cup of fresh or frozen berries (if you use fresh, you will need to add ice for a thicker shake), half a frozen banana (If you slice it before you freeze it, it chops up more easily), one serving of soy or whey protein powder. Blend at the liquefy or chop ice setting.

Another option is to use tofu instead of the powder. It makes the shake very smooth. And since tofu takes on the flavor of whatever it's prepared with, you don't get any of that chalky protein shake taste.

Lunch

Pizza Dough

A 1 pound recipe makes one medium thin 12" pizza.

_ cup warm water
3 _ tsp. olive oil
1 _ whole grain non-enriched flour
1 tsp. sea salt
1 tsp. honey
1 tsp. dry yeast
1 tsp. dried Italian seasoning

Add all ingredients to bread pan in order given. Set your bread machine settings to "pizza dough". Walk away and leave machine to do all the work. Or, add all ingredients in a small mixing bowl in order given. Using a fork, whisk until dough is separated from sides of bowl. Take the dough out of bowl and form a ball with it. Knead ten times or until dough is smooth. Place back in bowl. Cover with plastic wrap. Set in warm place for 20 minutes or until dough is swollen. Remove from bowl and place dough on a lightly cornmeal-dusted pizza stone. Create pizza of your desire. Serve and be blessed.

Mom on the Run Tip: Make a double portion. When dough is done rising, divide into two portions. Remove one to pizza stone, if using immediately. Or, place in bowl greased with olive oil, turn dough over to coat it, cover with plastic wrap and refrigerate until ready to use.

Tuna Wrap

>   1 can tuna, drained
>   1 cup mayonnaise, more or less as per
>   your taste
>   _ cup chopped celery
>   Green leaf lettuce, washed and dried (about
>   4 leaves)

Mix tuna, mayonnaise and celery to taste. Spoon about one fourth of mixture into lettuce leaf. Wrap leaf to close and eat!

Roast Beef Wrap

>   Healthy whole wheat tortillas in any flavor
>   (I like the garlic and pesto)
>   Roast beef, sliced thin
>   Provolone cheese, sliced
>   Canola oil (or other organic) mayonnaise
>   Green leaf lettuce, washed and dried

Spread a thin layer of mayonnaise on an open tortilla. Layer roast beef slice, provolone slices, and green leaf lettuce. Wrap tortilla to close and eat!

Breaded Chicken Nuggets

(One large chicken breast will serve 2-3 small children.)

Boneless, skinless chicken breast, diced
Organic bread crumbs
Pat butter
Ranch dressing (made with organic may-
onnaise and either milk or buttermilk)

Put bread crumbs in a paper or plastic bag. Add diced chicken breast. Close bag and shake to cover chicken. Melt butter in skillet over medium heat. Add chicken to pan. Keep turning to brown. Cook completely, about 5 minutes. Serve with ranch dressing and carrot sticks.

Main Dishes

Halibut

> 2 lbs. halibut (about 5-6 portions)
> 2 tbsp. olive oil
> 2 tsp. fresh chives
> _ tsp. pepper
> 1 lemon halved
> 1 _ lb. asparagus spears, trimmed
> 1 clove garlic, crushed
> 1 pinch of sea salt

Preheat oven or grill to 350˚F. Remove halibut from its packaging, rinse in cold water. Pat dry. Place halibut on long piece of aluminum foil. Squeeze one half of lemon onto halibut. Brush fish halibut with olive oil. This locks in moisture. Top with chives and pepper. Slice other half of lemon into coins and place on halibut. Place asparagus spears in separate aluminum foil from halibut. Add two tablespoons of water and fresh crushed clove of garlic and sprinkle with sea salt. Gather the aluminum foil length wise into center of halibut and asparagus. Fold down. Place on grill or in oven side by side. Bake until halibut is opaque throughout, about 20 to 25 minutes. Bake asparagus to liking. The crisper it is the more nutrients it keeps. Remove from foil. Serve and be blessed!

Salmon and Wild Rice

>2 lbs. salmon (about 5-6 portions)
>2 tbsp. olive oil
>2 tbsp. honey
>1 lemon, halved
>A pinch of sea salt if desired

Preheat oven or grill to 350' F. Prepare wild rice according to instructions on outside of package. Remove salmon from its packaging, rinse in cold water. Pat dry. Place salmon on long piece of aluminum foil. Squeeze lemon over salmon. Brush with olive oil. This locks on moisture. Top with honey, sliced lemon, and a pinch of sea salt. Gather aluminum foil length wise into center of salmon. Fold down. Place on grill or in oven. Bake until salmon is opaque throughout. About 20-25 minutes. Remove from foil. Serve and be blessed.

Wild rice tip: For more taste, substitute water with equal parts of chicken broth. (homemade broth preferred)

Tilapia

If tilapia is frozen, defrost in refrigerator.

Brush both sides of tilapia with olive oil. Place tilapia on broiling pan. Sprinkle seasoning of choice. (Try a lemon pepper or lime pepper mix.) Broil for 4 minutes. Tilapia is done when it is opaque and flakes with a fork. Serve with a garden salad or your favorite steamed vegetables.

Orange Roughy

If orange roughy is frozen, defrost in refrigerator.

Place orange roughy on broiling pan. Place thin butter shavings on orange roughy. Sprinkle with paprika. Broil for 6 minutes, turn and broil for 4-6 more minutes. Orange roughy is done when it is opaque and flakes with a fork.

Barbecue Chicken Pizza

      Pizza crust from bread recipes
      1 cup barbecue sauce (no sugar added)
      2 cup grilled or baked chicken, cubed
      1 cup shredded Monterey jack cheese
      1 cup cheddar cheese
      1 cup chopped green bell pepper (and/or
         red and yellow bell pepper)

      Preheat oven to 350'F. Roll pre-prepared dough onto cornmeal-dusted pizza stone. Brush with barbecue sauce. Top with meat, vegetables, and cheeses. Place in mid-oven and bake for 30-35 minutes. Take out of oven. Let stand 5 minutes. Slice.

Turkey Breast and Veggie Pizza

A pinch of yellow corn meal (not enriched)
1 lb. pizza dough
1 8oz. can tomato sauce (no sugar added)
1 cup diced turkey breast
_ cup sliced zucchini
_ cup sliced yellow bell pepper
_ cup diced Roman tomato
_ cup diced avocado
2 cups mozzarella cheese

Preheat oven to 350°F. Roll pre-prepared
dough onto cornmeal-prepared pizza stone. Brush
with tomato sauce. Top with turkey, zucchini,
tomato, avocado and cheese. Place in mid-oven
and bake for 30-35 minutes. Take out of oven. Let
stand 5 minutes. Slice. Serve and be blessed!

Soy Garlic Chicken

>4 boneless, skinless chicken breasts
>Pat of butter
>Soy sauce to taste
>Garlic powder to taste

Melt one pat of butter in a skillet over medium heat. Rinse chicken and pat dry. Place chicken in buttered skillet. Sprinkle with garlic powder. Cook for 6 minutes. Turn, cook for 4-6 more minutes. If chicken is particularly thick, cover skillet while cooking. Add soy sauce for last minute of cooking. Serve with rice, pasta, or favorite steamed vegetables.

Sautéed Vegetables

>2 zucchini, sliced
>2 carrots, slivered
>2 tbsp. olive oil
>1 clove garlic, pressed
>A pinch of sea salt if desired

Place olive oil in large skillet. Place large skillet over high heat. Add vegetables, garlic and salt. Stir. Cook until edge of zucchini is brown (approx 3 minutes). Turn to medium heat, cover and let stand for 5 minutes, stirring vegetables at 2 _ minutes. Remove from heat. Serve with main dish and be blessed!

Fresh Fruit Salad
(The kids love this one!)

Large red delicious apples
Bananas
Strawberries
Grapes, red or green
Honey dew melon
Cantaloupe
Lemon juice

Cut up the fruit; let the kids help if they're old enough. Lightly sprinkle the apple slices with lemon juice to keep them from browning. Toss together and serve.

Tropical Fruit Salsa

> _ cup fresh sliced pineapple
> 1 banana, sliced and quartered
> _ cup kiwi, peeled, sliced and quartered
>   (1-2 kiwi's)
> _ cup red or green pepper, seeded and
>   chopped
> 2 green onions, thinly sliced
> 2 tbsp. fresh cilantro, snipped
> 1 lime, sliced in half and squeeze juice
>   from each half

Add all ingredients into a bowl. Stir. Refrigerate until chilled. Serve with corn chips for a snack.

Mom on the Run Tip: Make double portions and serve for dinner over grilled chicken, turkey or your favorite fish. It's delicious!

Notes

For information on hormone and anti-aging please contact Dr. David Korn, (480) 354-6700 (LWBC member).

For a complete copy of "The Health Triune" or chiropractic care and information please contact Dr. Matt Mannino (LWBC member).

For scriptures and confessions please refer to *Confessing God's Word* by Pastor Maureen Anderson.

Bibliography

Balch, James F. and Phyllis A. *Prescription for Nutritional Healing*. Avery Publishing Group, Inc. Garden City Park, New York. 1990.

Foster, Colman R. *Flexibility Training and Aerobic Fitness for the 40+ Generation*.

Mannino, Matt. *The Health Triune*.

Meyerowitz, Steve. *Juice Fasting & Detoxification*. Book Publishing Company. Summertown, Tennessee. 2002. 154 pgs.

Featured Products by Winword Authors:

Dr. C. Thomas Anderson
Pastor Maureen Anderson
Scot Anderson

Making Impossibilities Possible

Making Your Marriage a Love Story

Confessing God's Word

Wisdom Wins 1

Wisdom Wins 2

Are You Spirit Led or Emotionally Driven?

Me, My Country, My God

More Than A Dad

More Than A Dad Audio Book

Now That I'm Saved

To order or for more information,
visit Winword Publishing House online at:

www.winwordpublishing.com

Or contact us at:
480-985-6156

Winword
publishing house